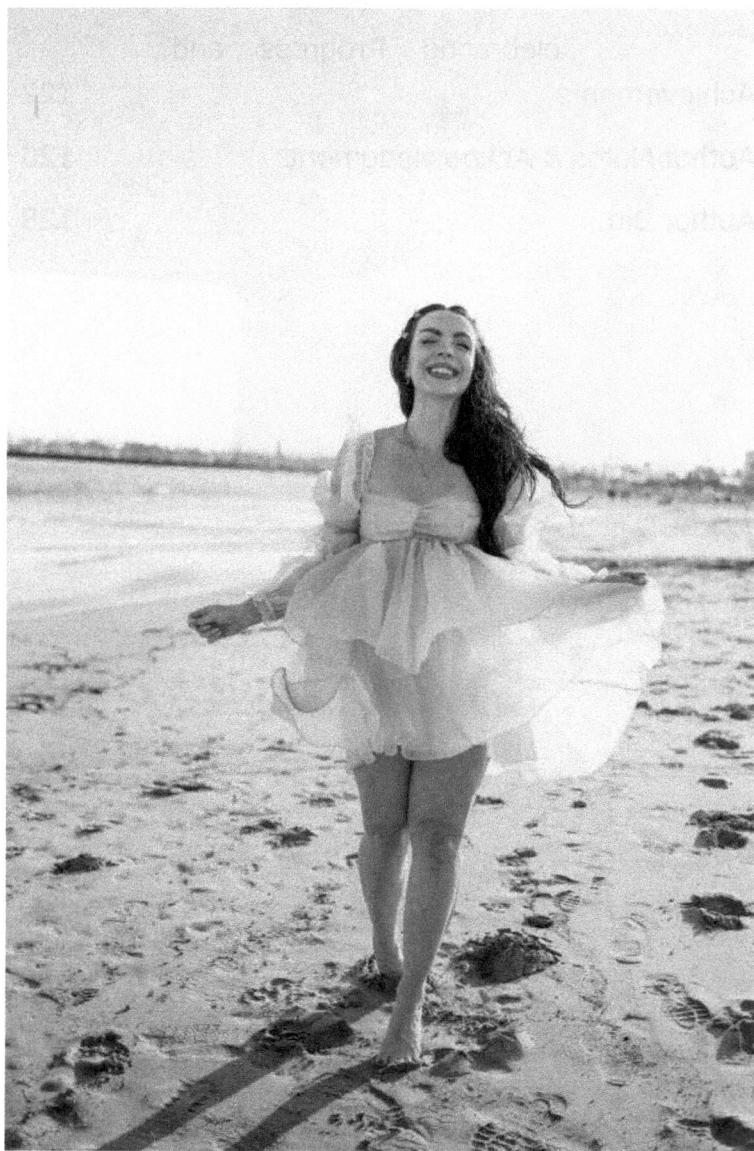

ISBN 978-1-998740-07-9 (Paperback)
ISBN 978-1-998740-08-6 (eBook)

Printed and bound in USA
Published by Loons Press

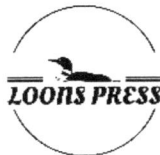

LOONS PRESS

Table Of Contents

Chapter 1

Understanding Asperger's Syndrome

Definition and Overview

Asperger's syndrome, now classified under the broader term of Autism Spectrum Disorder (ASD), is a neurodevelopmental condition characterized by challenges in social interaction, communication, and restricted or repetitive behaviors.

Individuals with Asperger's may exhibit a range of cognitive abilities, often possessing average or above-average intelligence. Understanding this condition is crucial for families and loved ones, as it provides insight into the unique experiences and challenges faced by those on the spectrum.

Recognizing that Asperger's is not a disease but a different way of processing the world can foster a more compassionate approach to support.

People with Asperger's often struggle with social cues and understanding the nuances of interpersonal relationships. This difficulty can manifest in various ways, such as challenges in making eye contact, interpreting body language, or engaging in small talk.

While they may desire social connections, the means to achieve these connections can feel overwhelming. Family members must recognize these hurdles, as patience and understanding are vital in creating an environment that encourages open communication and emotional expression.

Communication styles may also differ significantly for individuals with Asperger's. Many prefer direct, literal language and may find idioms or sarcasm confusing. This can lead to misunderstandings or frustration in conversations. Families should aim to adopt clear and straightforward communication methods, fostering an atmosphere where questions and clarifications are welcomed. Additionally, learning how to express emotions clearly can be beneficial for both parties, allowing for more effective interactions and reducing the potential for conflict.

In terms of routines and behaviors, individuals with Asperger's often thrive on predictability and structure. Changes in routine can be particularly challenging, leading to anxiety or meltdowns. Family members can help by providing a stable environment and preparing their loved ones for any changes in advance.

Visual schedules, checklists, and regular routines can assist in minimizing anxiety and enhancing a sense of security. Understanding the importance of these structures can empower families to create a supportive atmosphere that nurtures their loved one's strengths.

Finally, it is essential for families to recognize the strengths and talents often associated with Asperger's. Many individuals on the spectrum have exceptional focus, attention to detail, and expertise in specific areas, which can lead to unique contributions in various fields. Encouraging these strengths, rather than solely focusing on challenges, can build confidence and self-esteem.

Families can support their loved ones by celebrating their achievements, engaging in their interests, and fostering opportunities for them to shine. This positive reinforcement not only strengthens relationships but also promotes personal growth and fulfillment.

Characteristics of Asperger's

Individuals with Asperger's syndrome, now recognized under the broader category of Autism Spectrum Disorder (ASD), exhibit a range of distinct characteristics that can influence their social interactions, communication, and behavior. One of the most notable features of Asperger's is a marked difference in social communication.

Those with Asperger's may struggle to interpret social cues, such as body language and tone of voice, which can lead to misunderstandings in social situations. They often have difficulty initiating and maintaining conversations, which can make socializing challenging and may result in feelings of isolation.

Another characteristic common among individuals with Asperger's is a tendency towards intense focus on specific interests or hobbies. This intense focus can manifest in extensive knowledge about particular subjects, sometimes becoming a source of pride and achievement.

While this passion can lead to expertise in areas such as science, technology, or art, it may also result in challenges when individuals find it difficult to engage in topics outside their areas of interest. Family members can support their loved ones by encouraging a balance between their passions and exploring new activities together.

Sensory sensitivities are also prevalent in individuals with Asperger's. Many experience heightened or diminished responses to sensory stimuli, including sounds, lights, textures, and smells. For instance, a loud environment might be overwhelming, while certain fabrics may cause discomfort.

Understanding these sensory sensitivities is crucial for family members, as creating a comfortable environment can significantly enhance their loved ones' quality of life. Simple adjustments, such as providing noise-canceling headphones or creating a quiet space at home, can make a noticeable difference.

Repetitive behaviors or routines are another characteristic often associated with Asperger's. Individuals may engage in specific rituals or exhibit repetitive movements, such as hand-flapping or rocking. These behaviors can serve as coping mechanisms during times of stress or anxiety.

Family members should approach these behaviors with empathy and patience, recognizing that they may provide comfort or stability in an otherwise unpredictable world. Establishing a structured routine can help create a sense of security for individuals with Asperger's.

Lastly, emotional regulation can be a significant challenge for those with Asperger's. Many struggle to identify and manage their emotions, leading to heightened anxiety or frustration in social situations. This difficulty can also affect interpersonal relationships and daily functioning. Family members can play a vital role in helping their loved ones develop emotional awareness and coping strategies.

Encouraging open communication about feelings and providing tools for emotional expression, such as journaling or art, can foster greater emotional understanding and support healthier interactions with others.

Common Misconceptions

One of the most prevalent misconceptions about individuals with Asperger's is that they lack empathy. Many people believe that those on the spectrum are unable to understand or share the feelings of others.

However, research indicates that individuals with Asperger's can experience deep emotions and can empathize, though they may express it differently. They might struggle to interpret social cues or nonverbal communication, which can lead to misunderstandings.

It's essential for families to recognize that lack of eye contact or unusual responses do not equate to a lack of caring or emotional depth.

Another common myth is that individuals with Asperger's are uninterested in social interactions. While many may find socializing challenging, it does not mean they do not desire meaningful relationships. Some individuals may experience social anxiety or feel overwhelmed in group settings, leading to avoidance behaviors.

Families can play a crucial role by creating safe environments for social interaction and encouraging their loved ones to engage at their own pace. Understanding that the desire for connection exists, even if it's not always evident, is vital in offering appropriate support.

People often assume that Asperger's is a childhood disorder that one outgrows. This misconception can lead to significant misunderstandings about the lifelong nature of the condition. While early intervention and support can help individuals develop essential skills,

Asperger's does not simply disappear with age. Adults with Asperger's may continue to face challenges in social situations, employment, and relationships. Family members should be aware that ongoing support and understanding are necessary throughout their loved one's life to help them navigate the complexities of adulthood.

There is also a tendency to stereotype individuals with Asperger's as being exceptionally gifted in specific areas, such as mathematics or music. While some may indeed possess extraordinary talents, others may struggle academically or have different interests. This stereotype can pressure individuals who do not fit the mold, leading to feelings of inadequacy.

It is important for families to celebrate the unique qualities of their loved ones without imposing expectations based on societal stereotypes, thus fostering a sense of acceptance and self-worth.

Lastly, many people mistakenly believe that individuals with Asperger's are solely defined by their condition. This reductionist view overlooks the diverse identities, interests, and personalities that individuals possess. Families should focus on nurturing the whole person rather than solely identifying them by their diagnosis.

Encouraging hobbies, passions, and individual strengths allows those with Asperger's to thrive and be seen as complete individuals. Emphasizing their unique qualities can strengthen relationships and enhance their sense of belonging within the family and the broader community.

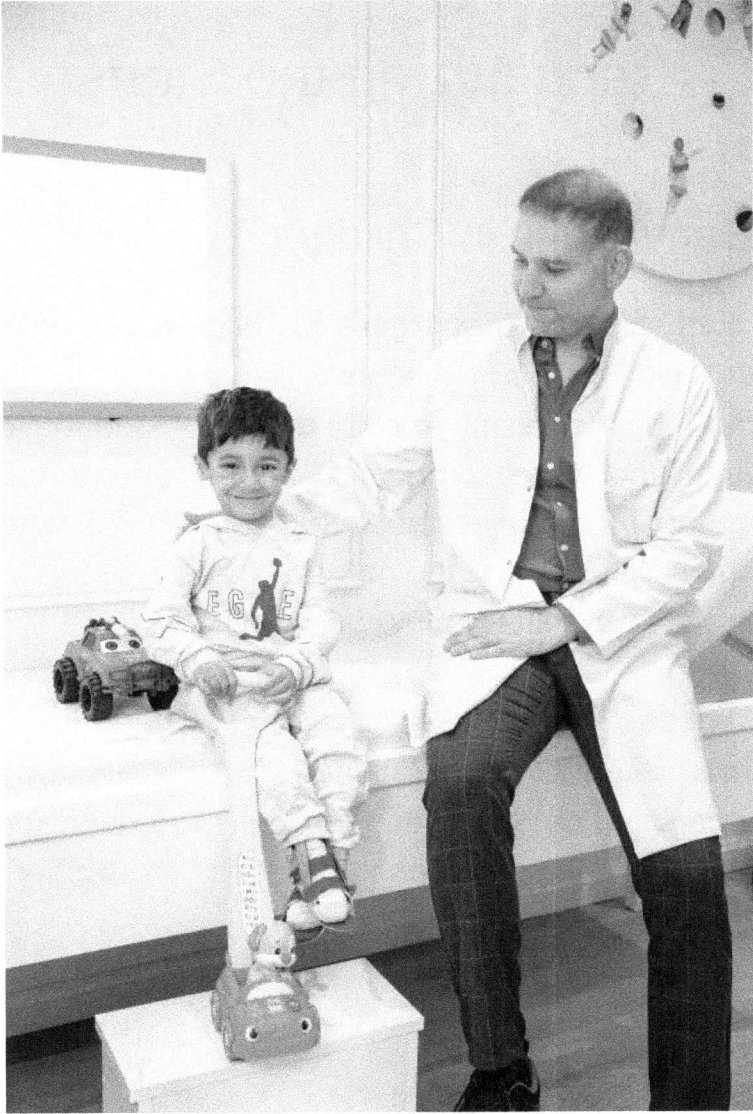

Chapter 2

Recognizing the Signs

Early Signs in Childhood

Early signs of Asperger's in children can often be subtle and may not become apparent until social interactions increase, typically during preschool years. Parents and caregivers may notice differences in communication styles, such as limited eye contact, difficulty in understanding nonverbal cues, or a preference for solitary play.

These behaviors can sometimes be misinterpreted as mere shyness or introversion, but they can indicate a deeper challenge with social engagement that is characteristic of Asperger's syndrome.

One of the most common early signs is a child's intense focus on specific interests or subjects. While many children develop strong interests, those with Asperger's may display an obsessive level of preoccupation.

This can manifest as extensive knowledge about a particular topic, often accompanied by a lack of interest in other activities or interactions. Recognizing this behavior can be vital for caregivers, as it may guide them in providing appropriate support and opportunities for socialization that incorporate these interests.

Language development can also serve as an indicator of Asperger's in young children. While children with Asperger's typically develop language skills at a normal rate, they may exhibit atypical patterns in their use of language. For instance, they may speak in a formal or pedantic manner, struggle with the nuances of conversational exchanges, or have difficulty understanding jokes and metaphors.

These communication challenges can lead to misunderstandings in social situations, making it crucial for families to foster an environment that encourages open dialogue and comprehension.

Another important aspect to consider is the child's response to sensory stimuli. Many children with Asperger's exhibit heightened sensitivity to sensory input, such as sounds, textures, or lights. This sensitivity may lead to overwhelming experiences in everyday situations, causing anxiety or frustration. Caregivers can support their loved ones by creating a sensory-friendly environment, allowing them to navigate their surroundings more comfortably and reducing potential stressors that may exacerbate their challenges.

Finally, observing a child's social interactions provides significant insight into their developmental trajectory. Children with Asperger's may struggle with forming friendships or understanding social norms, which can lead to feelings of isolation.

Early intervention through social skills training, playgroups, or therapy can be beneficial in helping them develop the necessary skills to build relationships. Families are encouraged to actively engage in these activities, fostering a supportive network that nurtures their loved one's social growth while reinforcing their unique strengths.

Signs in Adolescence and Adulthood

Signs of Asperger's Syndrome can manifest differently in adolescents and adults compared to children. During adolescence, individuals may experience heightened social pressures and expectations, which can exacerbate existing challenges.

Common signs include difficulties in navigating social situations, a tendency to engage in intense, focused interests, and struggles with understanding nonverbal cues. Adolescents may also exhibit anxiety related to social interactions or changes in routine, leading to withdrawal or frustration.

Recognizing these signs early can help families provide targeted support to facilitate smoother transitions during this critical developmental period.

In adulthood, the signs of Asperger's often evolve but can remain equally impactful. Many adults may continue to have difficulty with social interactions, finding it challenging to initiate or maintain conversations. They might misinterpret social norms, leading to awkwardness in professional and personal relationships.

Additionally, adults on the spectrum may develop coping mechanisms that allow them to mask their difficulties, which can sometimes result in increased stress or mental health issues. Understanding these signs is essential for family members who wish to foster a supportive environment that acknowledges and accommodates their loved one's unique experiences.

Communication challenges are prevalent throughout both adolescence and adulthood. Individuals with Asperger's may struggle with understanding figurative language, sarcasm, or humor, leading to miscommunication. They might prefer direct, clear communication, making it essential for family members to be mindful of how they express themselves.

By adopting a straightforward communication style and encouraging open dialogue, families can help their loved ones feel more comfortable expressing their thoughts and feelings. This approach not only aids in reducing misunderstandings but also strengthens familial bonds.

Emotional regulation is another area where signs of Asperger's can become apparent during adolescence and adulthood. Individuals may experience intense emotions but find it difficult to express or manage them appropriately.

This can lead to outbursts or meltdowns, particularly in overwhelming situations. Family members can support their loved ones by helping them identify and articulate their emotions, as well as by teaching coping strategies that promote emotional resilience. Creating a safe space for discussing feelings can greatly enhance emotional well-being and foster a sense of acceptance.

Ultimately, being aware of the signs of Asperger's in adolescence and adulthood enables families to provide informed and compassionate support. By recognizing the unique challenges faced at these stages of life, family members can advocate for their loved ones, ensuring they receive appropriate resources and opportunities for growth.

This proactive approach not only enhances the quality of life for individuals with Asperger's but also strengthens the overall family dynamic, promoting understanding and acceptance within the household.

Diagnosis and Assessment

Diagnosis and assessment of Asperger's syndrome, now referred to as part of the autism spectrum disorder (ASD), are essential processes for understanding the needs and strengths of your loved one. Early identification can significantly impact the support and interventions that can be provided, leading to better outcomes.

The diagnostic process typically involves a comprehensive evaluation that includes clinical assessments, interviews, and standardized tests designed to assess social communication, behavior patterns, and emotional functioning.

A qualified healthcare professional, often a psychologist or psychiatrist, will conduct the assessment. They will gather information from multiple sources, including the individual, family members, and educators. This multidimensional approach ensures that the diagnosis considers the individual's unique experiences and challenges.

It is crucial to be open and honest during this process, as the insights provided can greatly influence the understanding of your loved one's needs and how best to support them.

Following the initial assessment, a formal diagnosis may be made based on criteria outlined in the Diagnostic and Statistical Manual of Mental Disorders (DSM-5). This manual provides specific guidelines for identifying the various characteristics of ASD, including difficulties in social interactions, communication challenges, and restricted or repetitive behaviors.

Understanding these criteria can help families recognize the signs and better support their loved ones by tailoring their approaches to the specific challenges faced.

It is equally important to remember that a diagnosis is just the beginning of a journey. It opens the door to various resources, therapies, and interventions that can significantly enhance your loved one's quality of life.

Families should seek out information about available support services, educational resources, and community programs that specialize in ASD. Engaging with professionals who understand the nuances of Asperger's can empower families to develop effective strategies for communication and social interaction.

Lastly, ongoing assessment and reevaluation are vital as individuals with Asperger's grow and change over time. Regular check-ins with professionals can help identify new strengths and challenges, ensuring that support remains relevant and effective. By staying informed and engaged, families can foster an environment that encourages growth, understanding, and acceptance, ultimately leading to a more fulfilling life for their loved ones on the autism spectrum.

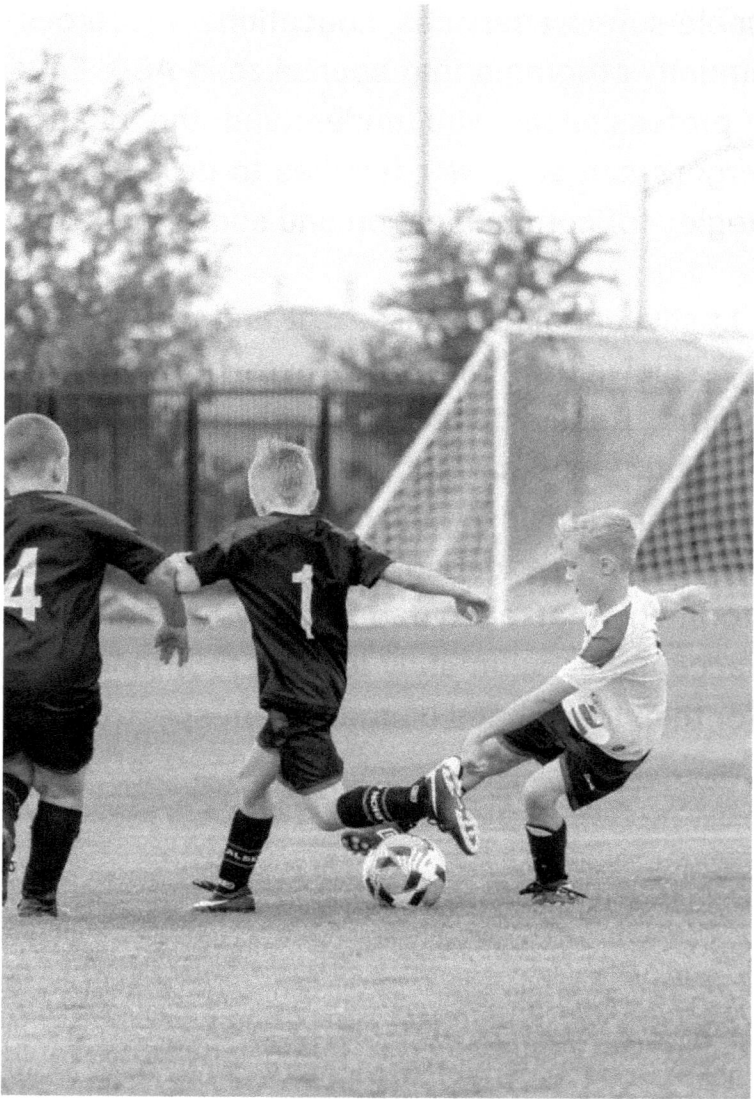

Chapter 3

Communication Strategies

Effective Communication Techniques

Effective communication techniques are essential for fostering understanding and connection with loved ones who have Asperger's. These techniques not only enhance interpersonal interactions but also help create a supportive environment where individuals feel valued and understood. One of the primary strategies is to use clear and direct language.

Individuals with Asperger's may struggle with interpreting figurative language or implied meanings, so it is beneficial to communicate in straightforward terms. Avoiding idioms, sarcasm, or ambiguous statements can prevent misunderstandings and facilitate better communication.

Non-verbal communication plays a significant role in interactions, particularly for those on the autism spectrum. While individuals with Asperger's may not always interpret non-verbal cues effectively, being aware of your own body language, facial expressions, and tone of voice is crucial.

Maintain an open posture and ensure that your facial expressions align with your words. This consistency helps convey sincerity and can make your loved one feel more secure and understood, even if they may not fully grasp all the non-verbal signals.

Listening actively is another vital component of effective communication. This involves not only hearing the words spoken but also understanding the feelings and intentions behind them. Encourage your loved one to express their thoughts and feelings, and provide them with your full attention. Nodding, maintaining eye contact, and using verbal prompts like "I see" or "Go on" can show that you are engaged in the conversation.

This approach fosters a safe space for open dialogue and encourages your loved one to share more openly, which can be particularly beneficial for those who may struggle with initiating conversation.

Establishing a routine can also enhance communication. Predictability can reduce anxiety for individuals with Asperger's, making it easier for them to engage in conversations. By scheduling regular times to talk about specific topics or simply check in with each other, you can create a comfortable structure. During these times, be sure to discuss any changes or upcoming events in advance, as this preparation can help your loved one feel more at ease and ready to communicate.

Lastly, being patient and empathetic is crucial in all interactions. Recognizing that communication may take longer or require more effort for your loved one can help you adjust your expectations and approach. When misunderstandings occur, try to remain calm and supportive rather than frustrated.

Acknowledge their feelings and validate their experiences, even if you do not fully understand their perspective. This patience and empathy will not only enhance communication but also strengthen your relationship, creating a more compassionate and understanding environment for both of you.

Non-Verbal Communication

Non-verbal communication plays a crucial role in human interaction, particularly for individuals with Asperger's syndrome. Understanding how non-verbal cues function can significantly enhance the ability of family members to connect with their loved ones. Non-verbal communication encompasses body language, facial expressions, gestures, posture, and even tone of voice.

For those on the autism spectrum, interpreting these cues can be challenging, which may lead to misunderstandings in social situations. Consequently, it is essential for families to learn how to recognize and adapt their own non-verbal communication to create an environment of support and clarity.

One key aspect of non-verbal communication is body language. While many people naturally pick up on subtle signals such as crossed arms or leaning away, individuals with Asperger's may struggle to interpret these gestures. Family members should be mindful of their body language when interacting with their loved one.

Open and relaxed postures can signal warmth and acceptance, whereas tense or closed postures might convey discomfort or disinterest. By being conscious of their own body language, family members can foster a more inviting atmosphere that encourages open dialogue and emotional connection.

Facial expressions are another vital component of non-verbal communication. Many individuals with Asperger's find it difficult to read or express emotions through facial cues. As a family member, it is helpful to communicate emotions clearly and explicitly, using both words and facial expressions.

For example, when discussing feelings, complementing verbal expressions with appropriate facial cues can help convey the intended message more effectively.

Additionally, families can practice recognizing different emotional expressions together, which can enhance their loved one's ability to understand and respond to others' emotions over time.

Gestures and tone of voice are also significant elements of non-verbal communication. Simple gestures, such as nodding or shaking one's head, can provide essential feedback during conversations. It is beneficial for families to use clear and consistent gestures to reinforce verbal messages.

Moreover, the tone of voice can greatly influence how a message is received. A warm and calm tone can alleviate anxiety and foster a sense of security for individuals with Asperger's, while a harsh or loud tone may lead to confusion or distress. Therefore, family members should pay attention to their tone, ensuring it aligns with their verbal messages to maintain clarity and support.

In summary, mastering non-verbal communication can significantly enhance the way families interact with their loved ones with Asperger's syndrome. By being aware of body language, facial expressions, gestures, and tone of voice, family members can create an environment that promotes understanding and connection.

As families practice these skills, they will likely notice improved communication and a stronger emotional bond with their loved ones, ultimately leading to a more supportive and harmonious family dynamic.

Encouraging Open Dialogue

Encouraging open dialogue is essential for fostering understanding and connection between individuals with Asperger's and their loved ones. Communication can often be a challenge, but creating an environment where open conversations are welcomed can significantly enhance relationships.

It is crucial for family members to approach discussions with patience and empathy, recognizing that individuals with Asperger's may communicate differently or may struggle with social cues. This understanding can set the stage for more meaningful interactions.

To promote open dialogue, it is beneficial to establish a safe space for conversations. This involves choosing a comfortable environment where the individual feels secure and less pressured. Family members should remind themselves to listen actively, giving their loved one the opportunity to express their thoughts and feelings without interruption.

Nonverbal cues, such as maintaining eye contact and nodding, can signal that the listener is engaged and values the speaker's contributions. This practice not only encourages the individual to share but also reinforces their confidence in communicating.

Additionally, it is helpful to ask open-ended questions that invite deeper responses rather than simple yes or no answers. Questions such as "How do you feel about that?" or "What do you think we should do next?" can stimulate discussion and provide insight into the individual's perspective.

It is essential to be mindful of the timing of these questions, ensuring that they are posed when the individual is receptive and comfortable. This approach can help in revealing their thoughts and emotions, which may otherwise remain unexpressed.

Another important aspect of encouraging open dialogue is to validate the feelings and experiences of the individual with Asperger's. Acknowledging their emotions, even if they differ from your own, can create a sense of acceptance and understanding. Statements such as "I can see that this is important to you" or "Your feelings are valid" can promote trust and openness. When individuals feel that their emotions are recognized, they are more likely to engage in meaningful conversations and share their thoughts without fear of judgment.

Finally, it is vital to be consistent in practicing open dialogue. Regularly engaging in conversations can help to normalize the process and make it a part of everyday interactions. Family members should be proactive in checking in on their loved ones, providing opportunities for them to share their feelings and thoughts.

This consistency not only strengthens relationships but also fosters a deeper understanding of the unique experiences faced by individuals with Asperger's. In this way, open dialogue becomes a cornerstone of support, enabling families to navigate the complexities of communication together.

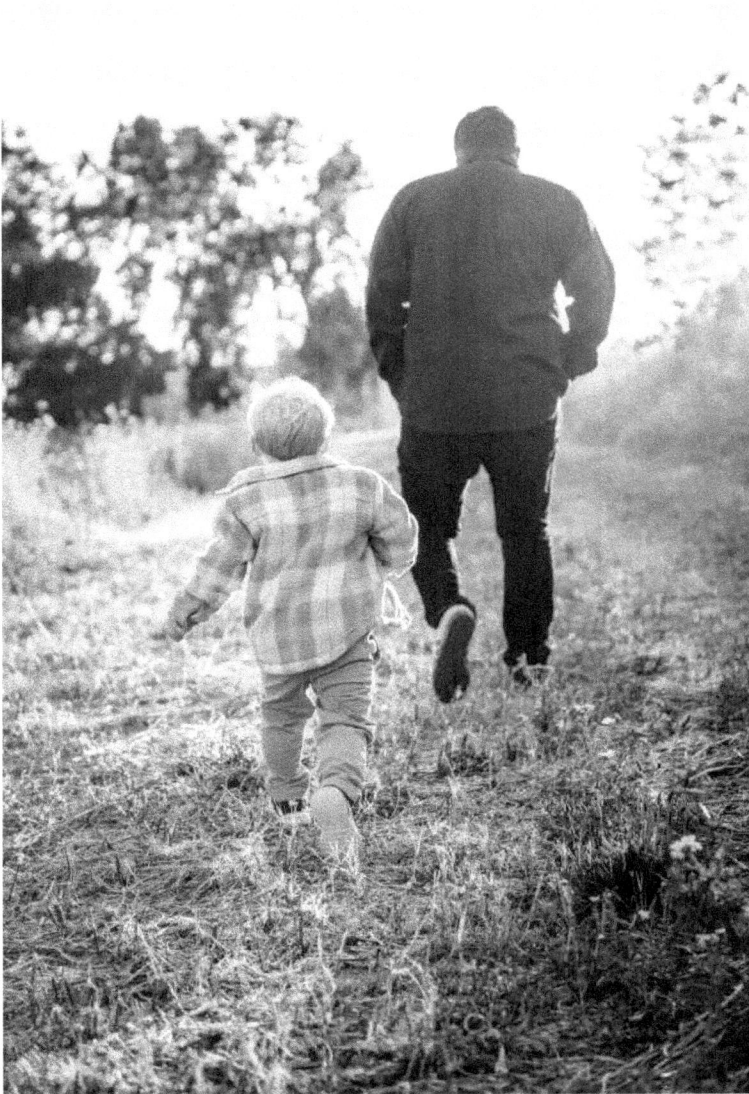

Chapter 4

Building Relationships

Understanding Emotional Needs

Understanding the emotional needs of a loved one with Asperger's is crucial for fostering a supportive and nurturing environment. Individuals on the autism spectrum often experience emotions differently and may struggle to identify, communicate, or manage their feelings. This can create a disconnect between them and their family members.

Recognizing these emotional needs is the first step in building a stronger relationship, as it allows families to respond more effectively to their loved one's experiences and challenges.

One key aspect of emotional needs for individuals with Asperger's is the need for predictability and routine. Many people on the spectrum thrive in structured environments where they can anticipate what will happen next.

Sudden changes or unexpected events can lead to anxiety and stress. Families can support their loved ones by establishing consistent routines and preparing them in advance for any changes. This not only helps to alleviate anxiety but also fosters a sense of security and stability, which is essential for emotional well-being.

Additionally, individuals with Asperger's may have difficulty expressing their emotions verbally. They might find it challenging to articulate feelings of sadness, frustration, or joy. As such, non-verbal cues become significant indicators of their emotional state.

Family members can learn to recognize these signals, which may include changes in behavior, body language, or withdrawal from social interactions. By being attuned to these non-verbal expressions, families can offer appropriate support and encouragement, helping their loved ones feel understood and valued.

Another important emotional need is the desire for acceptance and understanding. People with Asperger's often face social challenges, leading to feelings of isolation or exclusion.

It is essential for family members to create an inclusive atmosphere where their loved one feels safe to be themselves without fear of judgment. This can involve actively engaging in conversations about their interests, validating their feelings, and showing appreciation for their unique perspectives. When loved ones feel accepted for who they are, it significantly boosts their self-esteem and emotional resilience.

Finally, fostering independence while providing support is a delicate balance that addresses emotional needs. Encouraging a loved one with Asperger's to pursue their interests and develop social skills can enhance their sense of autonomy. However, it is important for families to remain available for guidance and assistance when needed.

By empowering their loved ones to take the lead in their own lives, families can help them build confidence and develop coping strategies for emotional challenges. This approach not only strengthens family bonds but also promotes overall emotional health for individuals with Asperger's.

Fostering Trust and Connection

Fostering trust and connection with a loved one who has Asperger's can significantly enhance communication and strengthen relationships. Trust is built through consistency, understanding, and patience. It is essential to create an environment where your loved one feels safe and valued.

This can be accomplished by actively listening to their concerns, validating their feelings, and engaging in open dialogue. When they sense that their thoughts and emotions are respected, they are more likely to share their experiences and challenges, leading to a deeper connection.

Establishing routines can also be a powerful way to foster trust. Individuals with Asperger's often thrive in structured environments where they know what to expect. By working together to create daily routines, family members can provide their loved ones with a sense of stability and predictability.

This not only reduces anxiety but also allows them to feel more secure in their interactions with family members. Consistent routines can serve as a foundation for communication, helping to build a trusting relationship over time.

Empathy plays a crucial role in nurturing connections with loved ones on the autism spectrum. Understanding their unique perspective and the challenges they face can help family members respond more effectively to their needs.

Taking the time to educate oneself about Asperger's can equip family members with the tools necessary to navigate social nuances and emotional responses. By demonstrating empathy, family members show their loved ones that they are not alone in their experiences and that their feelings matter.

Non-verbal communication is another vital aspect of fostering trust and connection. Many individuals with Asperger's may struggle with interpreting social cues, so it is important to be aware of your body language, facial expressions, and tone of voice.

Simple gestures, like maintaining eye contact or using a calm tone, can convey support and understanding. Additionally, encouraging your loved one to express themselves through alternative means, such as art or writing, can bridge communication gaps and foster a deeper connection.

Finally, patience is key in the journey of fostering trust and connection. Building a strong relationship with a loved one who has Asperger's may take time and effort. It is important to celebrate small victories and remain committed to the process, even when challenges arise.

Acknowledging progress, no matter how minor, can strengthen the bond between family members. By remaining patient and persistent, families can create a nurturing environment that promotes trust, understanding, and a lasting connection.

Social Skills Development

Social skills development is a crucial area of focus for individuals with Asperger's syndrome. These skills encompass a range of behaviors that facilitate effective interactions with others, including communication, understanding social cues, and building relationships.

For families supporting loved ones with Asperger's, understanding the nuances of social skills development can significantly enhance their ability to provide effective support. It is essential to recognize that individuals with Asperger's may face unique challenges in social situations, which necessitates tailored approaches to foster their social competencies.

One fundamental aspect of social skills development is the ability to recognize and interpret social cues. Individuals with Asperger's often struggle with non-verbal communication, such as facial expressions, body language, and tone of voice. These cues play a vital role in understanding the intentions and emotions of others.

Families can assist their loved ones by engaging in role-playing exercises that emphasize these non-verbal signals. By practicing in a safe environment, individuals can develop greater awareness and learn to respond appropriately in real-life situations, ultimately improving their interactions with peers and family.

Another important area is the development of conversation skills. Initiating and maintaining conversations can be particularly challenging for those with Asperger's. They may find it difficult to know what topics to discuss or how to read the interest levels of others in a conversation. Families can help by encouraging their loved ones to practice conversations with them, using structured prompts and topics of mutual interest.

This practice can include discussing current events, hobbies, or family activities, which can help build confidence and competence in conversational exchanges.

Building friendships is a vital component of social skills development that can greatly impact the overall well-being of individuals with Asperger's. However, forming and maintaining friendships often requires a different set of skills that may not come naturally. Families can support their loved ones by facilitating social interactions, such as arranging playdates or group activities where they can meet peers in structured settings.

Encouraging participation in clubs or community groups that align with their interests can also provide valuable opportunities for socialization, helping them to develop meaningful connections with others.

Lastly, it is essential to promote self-advocacy and self-awareness in the social skills development process. Individuals with Asperger's benefit from understanding their own strengths and challenges in social contexts. Families can engage in open discussions about social experiences, helping their loved ones to reflect on what went well or what could be improved. This reflective practice not only fosters self-awareness but also empowers individuals to advocate for themselves in social situations.

By encouraging them to express their needs and preferences, families can help their loved ones navigate social landscapes with greater confidence and resilience.

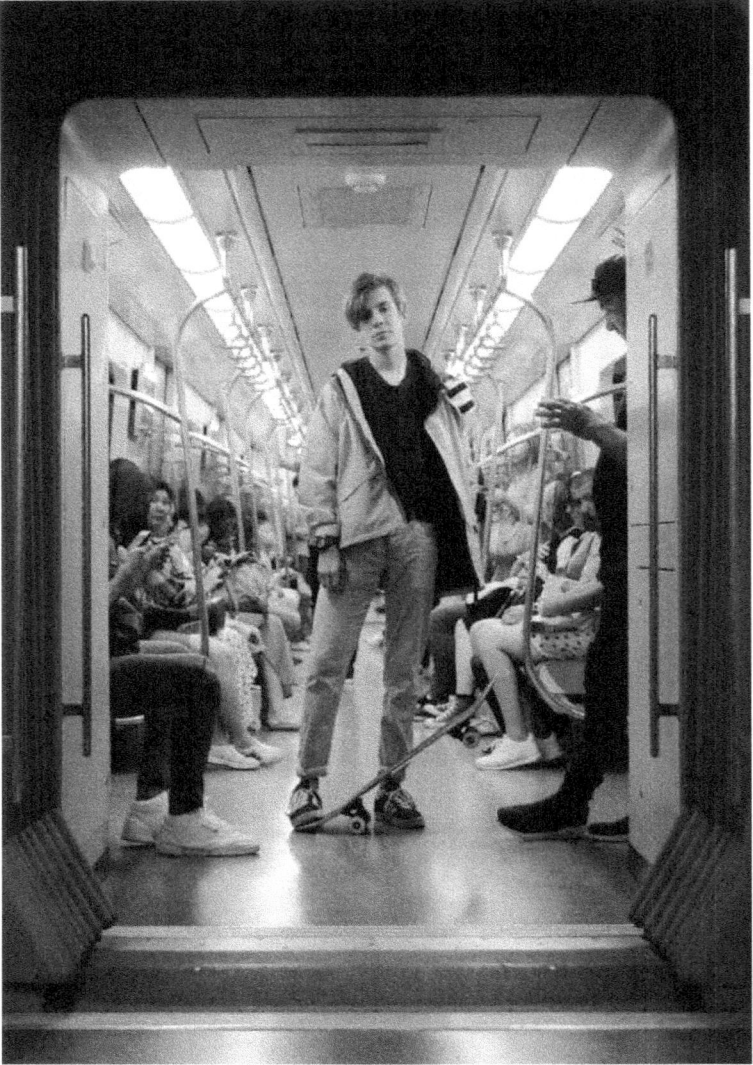

Chapter 5

Daily Life and Routines

Establishing a Structured Environment

Establishing a structured environment is crucial for supporting a loved one with Asperger's. Individuals on the autism spectrum often thrive in settings where routines are predictable and expectations are clear. By creating a structured environment, family members can help reduce anxiety and enhance the sense of security for their loved ones.

It is important to understand that what may seem like a minor adjustment to you can lead to significant improvements in their daily functioning and overall well-being.

One of the first steps in creating a structured environment is to establish consistent routines. This can include regular schedules for daily activities such as meals, chores, and leisure time. A visual schedule can be particularly effective, as it provides a clear representation of the day's events and helps your loved one anticipate what comes next.

By using visual aids, such as charts or calendars, you can make the routine more engaging and easier to follow. Consistency in routines not only fosters independence but also minimizes the stress associated with unexpected changes.

In addition to daily routines, it is essential to set clear expectations and rules within the household. Family members should communicate these expectations explicitly and reinforce them consistently. This can involve discussing household responsibilities, social interactions, and behavior in various settings. Providing a written list of rules can serve as a helpful reminder and reference for your loved one. When they understand what is expected of them, it can lead to improved compliance and a greater sense of empowerment.

Another vital aspect of a structured environment is creating a designated space for your loved one. This can be a quiet area where they can retreat when feeling overwhelmed or need time to recharge. Personalizing this space with their favorite items, such as books, toys, or sensory tools, can make it feel safe and comforting. Additionally, limiting distractions in the home, such as loud noises or chaotic environments, can help create a more conducive atmosphere for focus and relaxation.

Finally, it is important to involve your loved one in the process of establishing structure. Encourage their input on routines, rules, and personal spaces, which fosters a sense of ownership and collaboration.

By allowing them to participate in decision-making, you not only empower them but also increase their willingness to adhere to the established structure. Open communication about the benefits of a structured environment can lead to a more harmonious household and improved relationships among family members.

Creating Predictable Routines

Creating predictable routines is essential for individuals with Asperger's, as it fosters a sense of security and stability in their daily lives. Routines help reduce anxiety by providing clear expectations and minimizing surprises, which can be particularly challenging for those on the autism spectrum.

Establishing a consistent schedule allows loved ones to navigate their day with confidence, knowing what to expect at each moment. This predictability is not only comforting but also enhances their ability to focus on tasks without the added stress of uncertainty.

To create effective routines, it is important to involve your loved one in the planning process. Engaging them in discussions about their daily activities empowers them to express their preferences, which can lead to greater adherence to the established routine. Utilize visual aids such as charts, calendars, or checklists to illustrate the schedule.

These tools can serve as constant reminders of what comes next, making the routine more accessible and understandable. Additionally, consider including time for breaks and leisure activities, as this can help maintain motivation and prevent burnout.

Consistency is key when implementing routines. It is beneficial to stick to the same daily schedule as much as possible, as variation can lead to confusion and distress. If changes are necessary, communicate them in advance and explain the reasons behind them. This preparation can help mitigate anxiety and equip your loved one with strategies to cope with the unexpected. Over time, the individual will become accustomed to the routine, allowing them to adapt more easily to occasional changes.

Monitoring and adjusting routines is another critical component. Regularly assess how well the routine is working for your loved one. Are they feeling less anxious? Are they completing tasks more efficiently? Be open to feedback from them, as their insights can be invaluable in refining the routine.

If certain aspects are not working, it's okay to make changes. Flexibility within the framework of a routine can be beneficial, as it allows for growth and development while still providing the stability needed.

Finally, celebrate successes, no matter how small. Acknowledging achievements within the routine can boost self-esteem and reinforce positive behavior. Whether it's completing a task on time or successfully adapting to a minor change, recognizing these moments can enhance motivation and encourage your loved one to continue engaging with their routine. Creating predictable routines is not just about structure; it's about fostering a supportive environment where your loved one can thrive.

Managing Transitions and Changes

Managing transitions and changes can be particularly challenging for individuals with Asperger's, as they often thrive on routine and predictability. For families supporting a loved one with Asperger's, understanding the nuances of these transitions is essential.

Whether it's a change in school, a new job, or even a shift in family dynamics, recognizing the potential stressors involved can help families navigate these situations more effectively. Providing consistent support during these times can ease anxiety and facilitate smoother adjustments.

Establishing a clear communication strategy is key in managing transitions. Families should engage their loved ones in discussions about upcoming changes as early as possible. This allows individuals with Asperger's to process the information at their own pace.

Visual aids, such as calendars or checklists, can be beneficial in illustrating the timeline of the transition. Additionally, rehearsing scenarios or role-playing can help prepare them for what to expect, enabling them to feel more confident and less overwhelmed.

Creating a supportive environment is crucial during times of change. Familiarity can be comforting, so maintaining aspects of their routine that can remain unchanged is important. Families can work together to identify which elements of daily life provide stability and can be preserved amidst the transition.

Establishing a designated "safe space" at home, where the individual can retreat when feeling overwhelmed, can also provide a sense of security during these shifts.

Encouraging flexibility is another essential aspect of managing transitions. While routines are important, teaching loved ones to adapt to changes gradually can foster resilience. Families can implement small, manageable changes in their schedules to practice adaptability without causing undue stress. Positive reinforcement for successfully navigating minor changes can build confidence and prepare individuals for larger transitions in the future.

Lastly, it is vital for families to take care of their own well-being during these challenging times. Managing transitions can be emotionally taxing for caregivers and family members. Seeking support from local or online communities, as well as professional resources, can provide guidance and reassurance. By prioritizing self-care and maintaining open lines of communication, families can create a balanced approach that benefits everyone involved while supporting their loved one through transitions and changes.

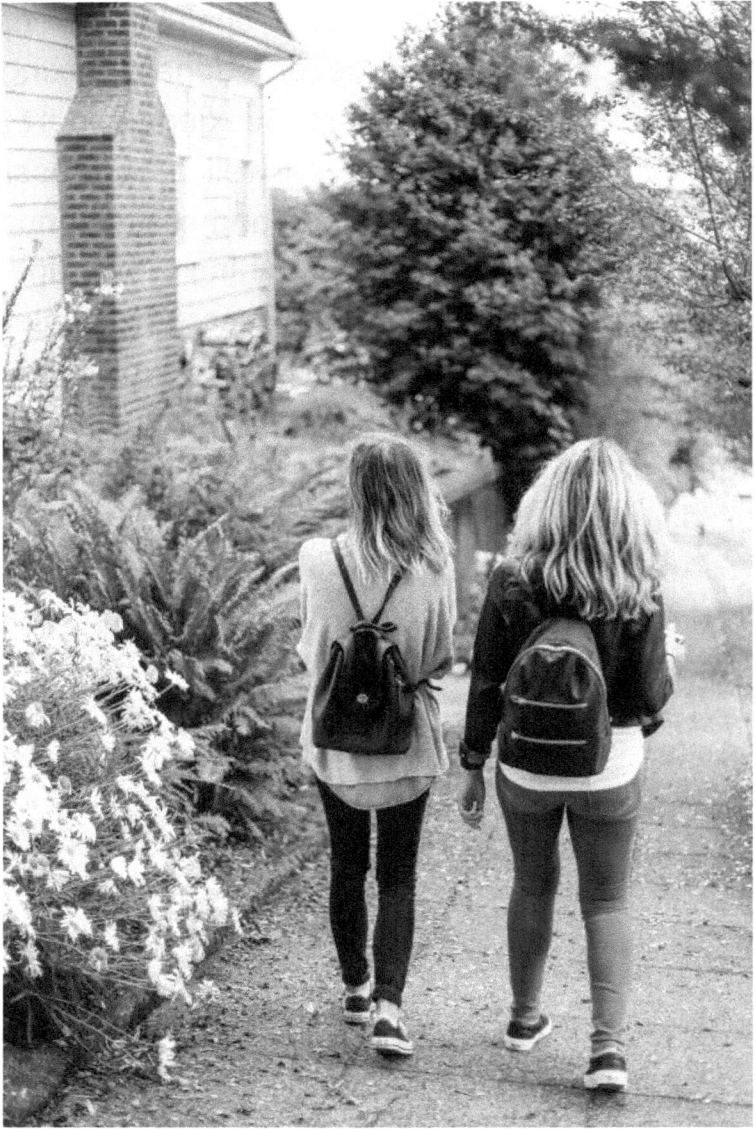

Chapter 6

Supporting Education and Career

Collaborating with Educators

Collaborating with educators is a crucial aspect of ensuring that loved ones with Asperger's receive the support they need in an academic setting. Parents and family members play a vital role in this collaboration, acting as advocates for their loved ones.

Building a strong relationship with teachers and school staff can lead to a more tailored educational experience that meets the unique needs of individuals with Asperger's. Open communication is key; by sharing insights about the individual's strengths, challenges, and preferred learning styles, family members can help educators create a more inclusive environment.

Understanding the school's resources and support systems is essential for effective collaboration. Many schools have special education teams, counselors, and psychologists who can provide additional assistance. Familiarizing yourself with the available programs can empower families to seek the right accommodations, whether it's an individualized education program (IEP) or a 504 plan.

These plans can outline specific strategies and resources, ensuring that the educational approach respects the individual's unique neurological profile and promotes their academic success.

Regular communication with educators helps in monitoring progress and addressing concerns promptly. Establishing a routine for meetings can keep everyone on the same page. It is beneficial to document observations about the loved one's behavior and academic performance to share during these discussions. This documentation can provide educators with valuable insights that inform instructional strategies and behavioral interventions.

By fostering an ongoing dialogue, families can ensure that adjustments are made as needed, allowing for a responsive educational experience.

In addition to direct communication with teachers, involving the loved one in discussions about their education can be empowering. Encouraging them to express their preferences and concerns can help educators understand their perspective. This involvement can also boost the individual's confidence and self-advocacy skills. When family members support their loved one in sharing their needs, it reinforces the importance of collaboration and respect for their autonomy in the learning process.

Finally, celebrating successes, no matter how small, can strengthen the partnership between families and educators. Positive reinforcement can motivate both the loved one and the teachers to continue their efforts. Recognizing achievements fosters a sense of community and shared purpose, which is essential for effective collaboration.

By working together, families and educators can create an environment that not only supports the educational needs of individuals with Asperger's but also promotes their overall well-being and development.

Navigating School Challenges

Navigating school challenges can be particularly daunting for individuals with Asperger's, as the educational environment often presents unique hurdles. These challenges can manifest in various ways, including difficulties with social interactions, sensory overload, and issues with communication.

Each child is different, so understanding the specific needs of your loved one is essential when addressing these obstacles. By equipping yourself with knowledge and strategies, you can play a vital role in helping them thrive in school settings.

One significant challenge faced by students with Asperger's is social interaction. Many children on the spectrum struggle to understand social cues and may find it hard to make or maintain friendships.

This can lead to feelings of isolation and anxiety, which can impact their overall academic performance. Encouraging social skills development at home through role-playing and discussing different scenarios can be beneficial. Additionally, collaborating with teachers to create opportunities for your loved one to engage with peers in structured environments can help foster these important skills.

Sensory sensitivities are another common issue that may arise in school. Many students with Asperger's experience heightened sensitivity to sounds, lights, and textures, which can create significant discomfort. It is crucial to communicate these sensitivities to school staff.

Working together to create a sensory-friendly environment, such as allowing the child to use noise-canceling headphones or having a designated quiet space to retreat to during overwhelming moments, can greatly enhance their comfort and focus throughout the school day.

Communication challenges often accompany Asperger's, and these can hinder a student's ability to express their needs or seek help when necessary. Encouraging open lines of communication between your loved one and their teachers can make a significant difference.

This may involve regular check-ins with educators to ensure they are aware of your loved one's communication style and preferences. Additionally, helping your loved one develop self-advocacy skills can empower them to express their concerns and needs more effectively, fostering a more supportive educational experience.

Finally, it is essential to advocate for your loved one within the school system. Familiarize yourself with special education resources and legal rights that can provide your loved one with the necessary accommodations. This may include Individualized Education Programs (IEPs) or 504 Plans that outline specific support tailored to their needs.

By actively participating in meetings and collaborating with educators, you can ensure that your loved one receives the appropriate resources and support to navigate school challenges successfully, ultimately paving the way for a more positive educational experience.

Workplace Accommodations

Workplace accommodations are essential for individuals with Asperger's, as they can significantly enhance their ability to perform effectively in their jobs. Understanding the unique challenges faced by individuals on the autism spectrum can help family members advocate for the necessary adjustments in the workplace.

These accommodations may include changes to the work environment, modifications in communication styles, or adjustments to job responsibilities that align better with the individual's strengths and preferences.

One common accommodation is providing a structured work environment. Many individuals with Asperger's thrive in settings that offer clear routines and predictable schedules. Employers can implement visual schedules or checklists to help employees manage their tasks effectively.

Additionally, minimizing sensory distractions in the workplace, such as excessive noise or bright lights, can further support productivity. Families can assist by suggesting these modifications during discussions with employers, emphasizing their loved one's needs.

Communication is another critical area where accommodations can make a substantial difference. Individuals with Asperger's may struggle with social interactions and non-verbal cues. Providing clear, written instructions and encouraging direct communication can help bridge this gap. Families can advocate for their loved ones by encouraging employers to adopt communication styles that are straightforward and unambiguous, ensuring that the individual understands expectations and can express any concerns without misunderstanding.

Job responsibilities can also be tailored to better suit the strengths of individuals with Asperger's. Many excel in specialized tasks that require focus and attention to detail. Families should work with their loved ones to identify these strengths and communicate them to potential employers.

This might involve suggesting roles that minimize social interactions or that allow for deep concentration on specific projects. By highlighting these capabilities, families can help create opportunities for success in the workplace.

Finally, ongoing support and open dialogue are vital in ensuring that workplace accommodations remain effective. As needs may change over time, it is essential for families to encourage their loved ones to maintain communication with their employers about any adjustments that might be necessary. Regular check-ins can help identify new challenges and solutions, fostering an environment where individuals with Asperger's feel empowered to advocate for themselves.

By working collaboratively with employers, families can create a supportive workplace atmosphere that enables their loved ones to thrive.

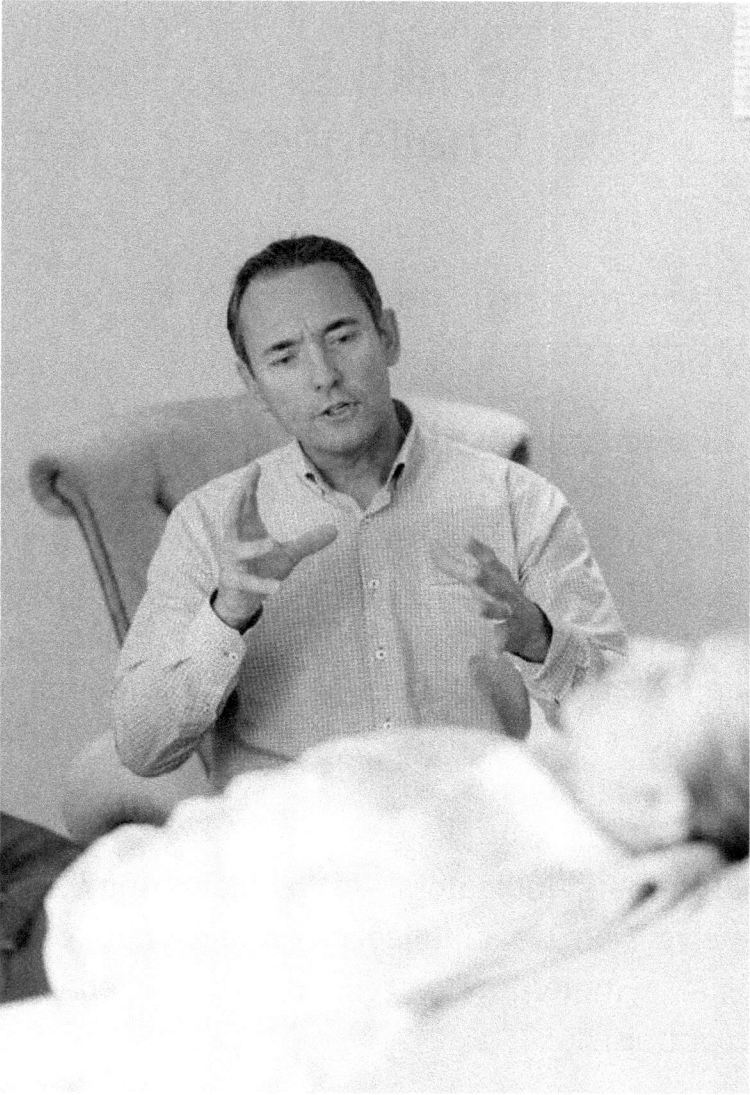

Chapter 7

Dealing with Emotional Challenges

Recognizing Anxiety and Depression

Recognizing anxiety and depression in loved ones with Asperger's can be challenging, yet it is crucial for providing effective support. Individuals with Asperger's may experience these mental health issues differently than those without the condition, often manifesting in unique behaviors and expressions. Understanding the signs and symptoms is the first step in offering meaningful assistance.

Common indicators of anxiety may include excessive worry, avoidance of certain situations, and physical symptoms like restlessness or changes in sleep patterns.

Depression might present as withdrawal from social interactions, a noticeable decline in interest in previously enjoyed activities, or expressions of hopelessness.

It is also essential to be aware of the subtler signs that may indicate anxiety or depression. Individuals with Asperger's often have difficulty articulating their feelings, which can lead to frustration and misunderstandings. Changes in routine or unexpected disruptions can exacerbate anxiety, resulting in irritability or meltdowns.

Observing changes in behavior or mood over time can provide significant insights. As a caregiver or family member, keeping a record of these changes can help in understanding patterns and triggers, making it easier to address concerns with the loved one or a professional. Communication plays a vital role in recognizing mental health struggles. Encourage open dialogues about feelings, fears, and frustrations. It is essential to create a safe space where your loved one feels comfortable expressing themselves without fear of judgment.

Simple, direct questions about how they are feeling can be effective. Moreover, using visual aids or writing down feelings might help in bridging the communication gap. Patience is key, as it may take time for them to articulate their emotions fully.

Another aspect to consider is the impact of sensory sensitivities on anxiety and depression. Individuals with Asperger's often experience heightened sensitivities to sensory inputs, which can contribute to feelings of overwhelm and distress. Loud noises, bright lights, or crowded spaces may trigger anxiety, leading to withdrawal or depressive symptoms.

Being attentive to these triggers and helping to create a conducive environment can significantly reduce stress levels. Small adjustments, such as providing noise-canceling headphones or creating a quiet space, can make a difference in their emotional well-being.

Finally, if you suspect that your loved one is struggling with anxiety or depression, it is essential to approach the situation with understanding and empathy. Encourage them to seek professional help if needed, and offer to assist in finding resources or accompanying them to appointments. Support groups and counseling can provide additional assistance and coping strategies.

By actively recognizing and addressing these mental health issues, you can foster a more supportive environment that enhances your loved one's quality of life and strengthens your relationship.

Coping Mechanisms and Strategies

Coping mechanisms and strategies are essential for families supporting loved ones with Asperger's. Understanding and implementing these strategies can create a more harmonious home environment and improve communication.

One effective approach is to establish clear routines. Individuals with Asperger's often thrive on predictability, so having a structured daily schedule can help reduce anxiety. This routine can include specific times for meals, activities, and downtime, providing a sense of security and stability.

Another important strategy is to focus on clear and direct communication. Individuals with Asperger's may struggle with understanding non-verbal cues or implicit messages.

As such, family members should aim to be explicit in their communication, using straightforward language and being mindful of tone and body language. This clarity can help prevent misunderstandings and foster a more open dialogue, allowing loved ones to express their thoughts and feelings more comfortably.

Creating a safe space for emotional expression is also vital. Family members should encourage their loved ones to share their feelings without fear of judgment. This can be achieved by actively listening and validating their emotions, even if they differ from the family's perspective.

Engaging in regular check-ins, where feelings and thoughts can be shared openly, can strengthen the bond between family members and provide individuals with Asperger's the reassurance that their experiences are valued.

In addition to communication and emotional support, teaching coping skills for managing anxiety and sensory overload can be beneficial. Techniques such as deep breathing, mindfulness, and sensory breaks can help individuals navigate overwhelming situations. Families can work together to identify triggers and develop personalized coping strategies that empower their loved ones. This proactive approach not only equips them with tools for managing stress but also fosters independence and self-advocacy.

Lastly, seeking professional support can enhance the effectiveness of these coping mechanisms. Therapists or counselors who specialize in Asperger's can provide tailored strategies and insights for both the individual and the family.

Participating in support groups can also connect families with others facing similar challenges, offering shared experiences and resources. By combining these strategies, families can create a supportive environment that promotes understanding, resilience, and growth for their loved ones with Asperger's.

Seeking Professional Help

Seeking professional help can be a crucial step in providing the best support for a loved one with Asperger's. Understanding that Asperger's is a spectrum condition means that every individual may require different types and levels of support.

Professionals such as psychologists, counselors, and occupational therapists have specialized training and experience that can greatly enhance the quality of life for both the individual with Asperger's and their family members. Engaging with these professionals can provide tailored strategies to address specific challenges and promote well-being.

One of the first steps in seeking professional help is to identify the specific needs of your loved one. This may involve observing their behavior, communication patterns, and social interactions. By pinpointing areas where they struggle, you can better articulate these concerns to a professional.

It is also important to consider the emotional needs of the family, as the challenges of supporting someone with Asperger's can take a toll on relationships. Family therapy may be beneficial in these cases, helping everyone to communicate openly and strengthen their bonds.

When looking for professionals, it is essential to find someone who has experience working with individuals on the autism spectrum. This can include searching for specialists who focus on social skills training, cognitive behavioral therapy, or sensory integration therapy.

Recommendations from trusted sources, such as pediatricians or school counselors, can be invaluable. Additionally, online resources and local support groups can provide insights and reviews of practitioners in your area, ensuring that you make an informed choice.

Once you have selected a professional, it is important to maintain open lines of communication. Establishing a collaborative relationship between your loved one, the professional, and family members can lead to more effective support strategies.

Regular check-ins can help assess progress and make necessary adjustments to the treatment plan. Be prepared to advocate for your loved one's needs and ensure that their voice is heard in the process. This partnership can empower both the individual and the family to work towards shared goals.

Lastly, remember that seeking professional help is not a sign of failure but rather a proactive step towards understanding and supporting your loved one. It can lead to improved coping strategies, enhanced social skills, and greater emotional resilience.

By embracing this process, families can foster an environment of growth and acceptance, enabling their loved ones with Asperger's to thrive. This journey may be challenging, but with the right professional guidance, it can lead to meaningful improvements in the quality of life for everyone involved.

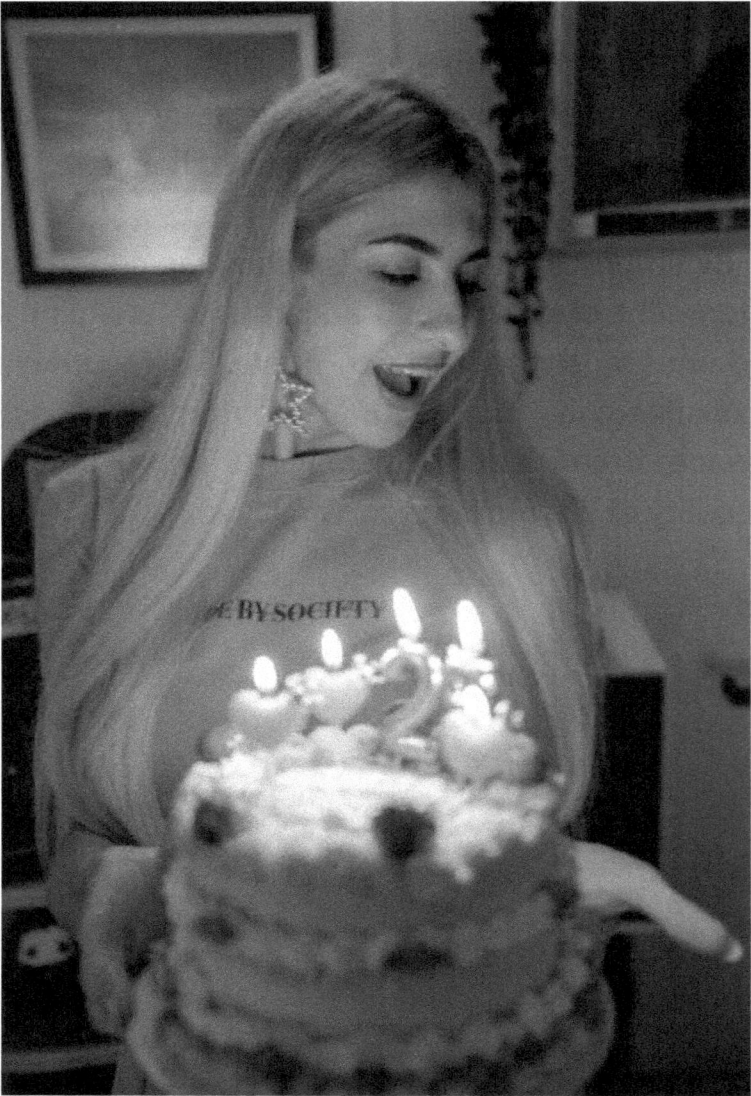

Lastly, remember that seeking professional help is not a sign of failure but rather a proactive step towards understanding and supporting your loved one. It can lead to improved coping strategies, enhanced social skills, and greater emotional resilience.

By embracing this process, families can foster an environment of growth and acceptance, enabling their loved ones with Asperger's to thrive. This journey may be challenging, but with the right professional guidance, it can lead to meaningful improvements in the quality of life for everyone involved.

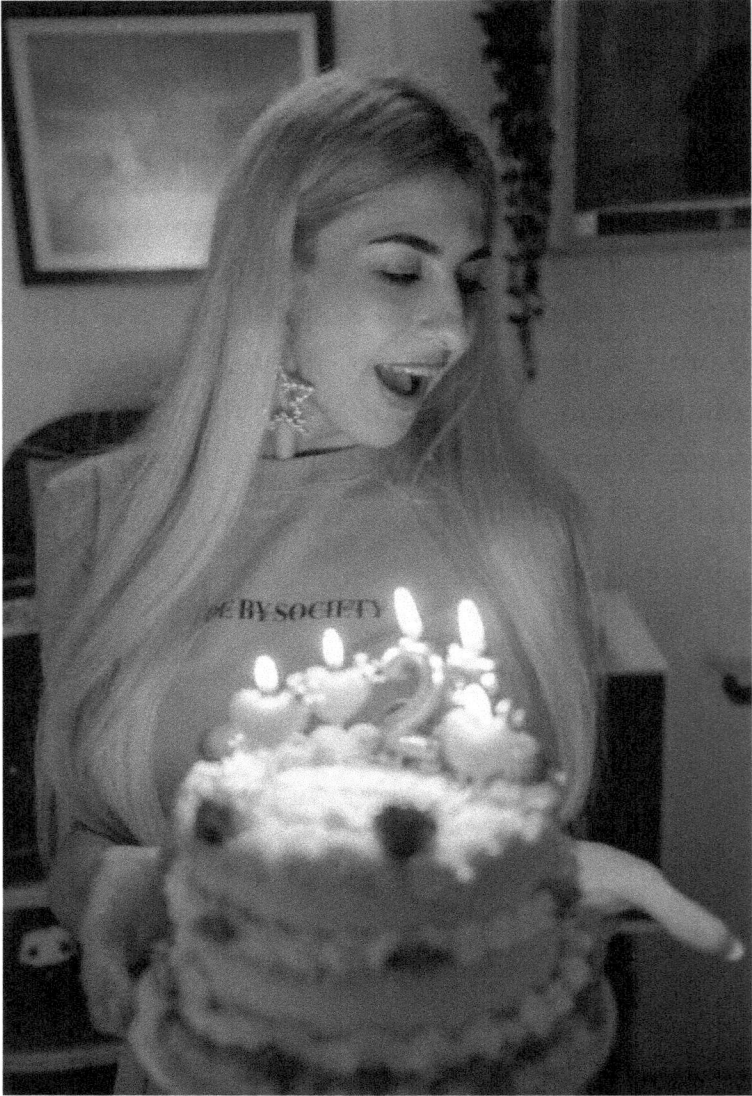

Chapter 8

Enhancing Independence

Life Skills Development

Life skills development is a crucial aspect for individuals with Asperger's, as it equips them with the practical abilities needed to navigate daily life more effectively. These skills encompass a wide range of areas, including personal care, social interactions, communication, and time management.

Families play a vital role in fostering these skills, providing the necessary support and encouragement to help their loved ones gain independence and confidence. By focusing on life skills, families can enhance the overall quality of life for individuals with Asperger's.

Personal care skills are foundational and form the basis for daily independence. Teaching your loved one how to manage personal hygiene, grooming, and dressing appropriately can significantly impact their self-esteem and social interactions.

Creating a structured routine can help reinforce these skills, allowing the individual to understand the importance of personal care. Visual schedules, checklists, and consistent reminders can be effective tools in this process. Celebrating small successes in personal care can motivate your loved one to continue developing these essential habits.

Social skills are another critical area of life skills development. Individuals with Asperger's often face challenges in understanding social cues and engaging in reciprocal conversations. Family members can assist by modeling appropriate social interactions and providing opportunities for practice in safe environments. Role-playing various social scenarios can help your loved one become more comfortable with different social situations.

Additionally, joining group activities or clubs that align with their interests can facilitate socialization and allow them to form meaningful connections with peers.

Communication skills are equally important and can significantly influence how individuals with Asperger's express themselves and understand others. Encouraging your loved one to articulate their thoughts and feelings can improve their overall communication abilities.

Utilizing tools such as visual aids, social stories, and technology can enhance their understanding and expression of complex ideas. Engaging in regular conversations about emotions and daily experiences can also promote better communication skills, helping them to articulate their needs and preferences effectively.

Time management is an often-overlooked life skill that can greatly affect the daily lives of individuals with Asperger's. Developing routines and schedules can help your loved one understand the concept of time and its importance in completing tasks.

Using timers, calendars, and reminders can assist in organizing their day-to-day activities. Teaching prioritization skills and breaking tasks into manageable steps can also alleviate feelings of overwhelm. By instilling effective time management strategies, families can empower their loved ones to navigate their responsibilities more efficiently and independently.

Encouraging Decision-Making

Encouraging decision-making in loved ones with Asperger's can foster independence and self-confidence. Individuals on the autism spectrum often benefit from structured guidance when faced with choices, as they might struggle with uncertainty or anxiety about potential outcomes. To support them effectively, it is crucial to create an environment where they feel safe to express their preferences and make decisions.

This can be achieved by providing clear options rather than overwhelming them with too many choices. Simplifying decisions into manageable parts can help them feel more in control and less intimidated.

One effective strategy is to engage in conversations that explore their interests and preferences. Asking open-ended questions can prompt them to think critically about what they want. For example, instead of asking, "Do you want to go to the park?" you could say, "What do you enjoy about going to the park?"

This approach encourages them to articulate their thoughts and feelings, allowing you to understand their perspective better. It also reinforces the idea that their opinions are valued, which is essential for building confidence in their decision-making abilities.

Incorporating visual aids can significantly enhance the decision-making process for individuals with Asperger's. Charts, diagrams, or even simple lists can help clarify options and potential outcomes. For instance, if they need to choose between two activities, you could create a visual comparison detailing the pros and cons of each option.

This method not only aids in understanding but also provides a tangible reference, making it easier for them to weigh their choices. Visual supports can serve as a bridge between abstract ideas and concrete decisions, facilitating a more informed choice.

Role-playing scenarios can also be a practical tool for encouraging decision-making. By simulating different situations, you can help your loved one practice how to approach decisions in a low-pressure environment.

For example, you could role-play a shopping trip where they must decide which item to buy. This hands-on experience allows them to navigate real-life situations while receiving guidance and feedback. Additionally, discussing the outcomes of these role-plays can help reinforce learning and improve their confidence in making similar decisions in the future.

Finally, it is important to celebrate their decision-making efforts, regardless of the outcomes. Positive reinforcement can motivate them to continue making choices and help them develop a sense of accomplishment.

Acknowledging their efforts – whether they made the right choice or learned from a mistake – reinforces that decision-making is a valuable skill. This support nurtures their ability to make choices independently, allowing them to grow and thrive as they navigate various aspects of life. By promoting a supportive atmosphere, you empower your loved one to embrace decision-making as a crucial part of their personal development.

Promoting Self-Advocacy

Promoting self-advocacy is a crucial aspect of supporting loved ones with Asperger's. Self-advocacy empowers individuals to understand their own needs, express their feelings, and make informed choices about their lives. It begins with fostering self-awareness, which involves helping them recognize their strengths, challenges, and preferences.

Encouraging open discussions about their experiences can help them articulate their thoughts more clearly. By creating a safe environment for dialogue, family members can assist in building the confidence needed for effective self-advocacy.

One of the key elements of promoting self-advocacy is teaching effective communication skills. Individuals with Asperger's may struggle with social cues and verbal expression, making it essential to provide them with the tools to communicate their needs. Role-playing different scenarios can be beneficial, as it allows them to practice how to express their feelings in various situations.

Additionally, using visual aids or written prompts can serve as helpful reminders for them when they encounter challenging interactions. The more comfortable they become with their communication skills, the more empowered they will feel to advocate for themselves.

Encouraging independence is another significant factor in self-advocacy. Family members can support their loved ones by gradually introducing them to situations that require decision-making and problem-solving. This might involve small tasks like planning their own meals, managing a budget, or setting personal goals.

By allowing them to take the lead in these areas, family members can foster a sense of ownership over their lives. Over time, this independence can translate into greater confidence in advocating for their needs and desires in broader contexts, such as school or work.

It is also essential to connect loved ones with appropriate resources and support systems. This can include local advocacy organizations, support groups, or even online communities tailored to individuals with Asperger's. Engaging with peers who share similar experiences can enhance their understanding of self-advocacy and provide a platform for sharing strategies.

Family members can assist by researching and presenting these opportunities, reinforcing the idea that they are not alone in their journey and that there are people and resources available to support them.

Finally, celebrating achievements, no matter how small, is vital in reinforcing self-advocacy. Acknowledging efforts to express needs or make decisions encourages continued growth and confidence. Family members should take the time to recognize these milestones, offering positive reinforcement and celebrating progress.

This practice not only boosts self-esteem but also reinforces the importance of self-advocacy as an ongoing journey. By consistently promoting self-advocacy, families can help their loved ones with Asperger's navigate their lives more effectively and become active participants in their own futures.

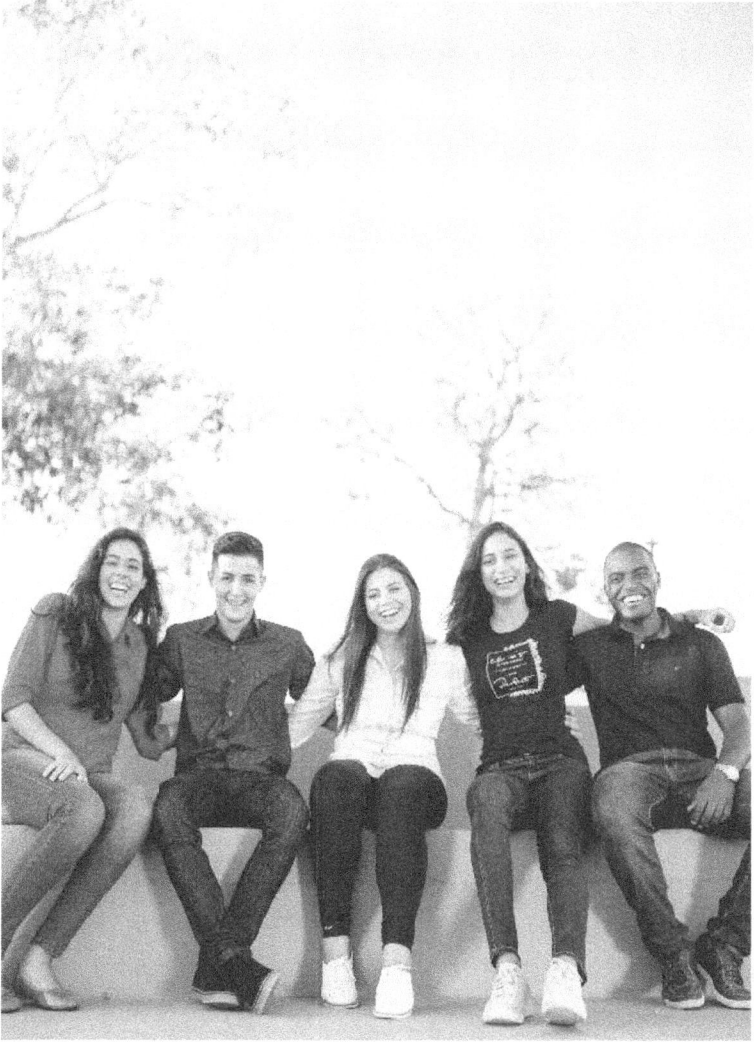

Chapter 9

Resources and Support Networks

Finding Local Support Groups

Finding local support groups can be a transformative step for families navigating the complexities of Asperger's syndrome. These groups serve as a vital resource for emotional support, information sharing, and communal strength.

By connecting with others who share similar experiences, family members can gain insights, coping strategies, and a sense of belonging that alleviates feelings of isolation. Many organizations, such as the Autism Society and local mental health agencies, maintain directories of support groups, making it easier to find a suitable match in your area.

When searching for local support groups, consider the specific needs of your family member with Asperger's. Some groups focus on particular age ranges, while others may cater to specific challenges, such as social skills development or behavioral issues. It is important to identify groups that align with your loved one's circumstances and your family's needs.

Additionally, some groups may be tailored for parents and caregivers, providing a space to discuss common challenges and share experiences while others may include individuals with Asperger's themselves, fostering an environment of mutual understanding.

In-person meetings can offer unique benefits, allowing for face-to-face interactions that can lead to stronger connections among participants. Local community centers, schools, and mental health clinics often host these gatherings. Attending meetings not only facilitates discussions but also provides opportunities for social interactions that can enhance your support network.

If in-person attendance is difficult due to geographic or logistical barriers, many organizations also provide virtual support groups, ensuring that everyone has access to the help they need.

When attending a support group for the first time, it can be helpful to approach the experience with an open mind and a willingness to share. Listening to the experiences of others can provide valuable perspectives and strategies that you might not have considered.

Engaging in discussions, asking questions, and expressing your own challenges can foster a sense of camaraderie and trust within the group. Remember that each person's journey is unique, and what works for one family may not work for another; however, collective experiences can illuminate new pathways to explore.

As you become more involved with local support groups, consider giving back to the community by volunteering or taking on a leadership role. This not only reinforces your commitment to supporting others but also helps you further develop your own understanding and advocacy skills.

By sharing your journey and the lessons learned, you can inspire and empower other families facing similar challenges. Ultimately, finding and participating in local support groups can significantly enhance your ability to support your loved one with Asperger's, creating a more informed and resilient family dynamic.

Online Resources and Communities

Online resources and communities have become invaluable tools for families supporting loved ones with Asperger's. The internet offers a wealth of information, ranging from educational articles and research studies to practical advice and personal stories.

These resources can help family members understand Asperger's better, providing insights into the challenges and strengths associated with the condition.

Websites dedicated to autism spectrum disorders often feature comprehensive guides, blogs, and forums where families can learn from experts and each other. Utilizing these resources can empower families to create a supportive environment for their loved ones.

One of the most beneficial aspects of online resources is access to virtual communities. These platforms allow families to connect with others who share similar experiences, fostering a sense of belonging and support. Social media groups, online forums, and dedicated websites can serve as safe spaces for discussing concerns, sharing strategies, and celebrating successes.

Engaging with these communities can alleviate feelings of isolation and provide reassurance that families are not alone in their journey. The shared experiences can also offer practical tips that have worked for others, which can be beneficial in day-to-day interactions.

In addition to community support, various online resources provide access to webinars, online courses, and workshops tailored to families of individuals with Asperger's. These educational opportunities can enhance understanding of the condition and offer strategies to improve communication and relationships.

Many organizations focused on autism provide free or low-cost training sessions that cover a range of topics, from social skills development to managing sensory sensitivities. Participating in these sessions can equip family members with the tools needed to navigate challenges more effectively.

Additionally, there are numerous blogs and podcasts dedicated to sharing personal experiences of living with Asperger's. These platforms can provide unique perspectives that might resonate with family members.

Hearing firsthand accounts from individuals on the spectrum can deepen understanding and empathy, allowing family members to relate more closely to their loved ones' experiences. These narratives can also highlight the strengths and unique talents of individuals with Asperger's, fostering a more balanced view of the condition.

Lastly, it is essential for families to approach online resources critically. Not all information found online is accurate or helpful. Families should prioritize reputable sources, such as established organizations and professionals in the field of autism.

Engaging with evidence-based materials can ensure that families are receiving the best possible guidance. By taking advantage of online resources and communities while remaining discerning, families can enhance their ability to support their loved ones with Asperger's effectively.

Professional Organizations

Professional organizations play a crucial role in providing resources, support, and advocacy for individuals with Asperger's syndrome and their families. These organizations often serve as a bridge between families and the wider community, offering valuable information about the condition, available services, and emerging best practices in care and support.

By engaging with these organizations, families can access a wealth of knowledge that can empower them to better understand and support their loved ones.

One of the most recognized professional organizations is the Autism Society, which offers a range of programs focused on education, advocacy, and community support. The organization provides resources that help families navigate the challenges associated with Asperger's syndrome, including information on treatment options, educational resources, and support groups. Families can benefit from the shared experiences of others in the community, gaining insights that can help them to create a supportive environment for their loved ones.

Another key organization is the National Autism Association, which focuses on safety and support for individuals with autism spectrum disorders, including Asperger's. They provide resources on safety planning, community awareness, and training for first responders.

By being informed about safety issues and having resources at hand, families can proactively address potential challenges and ensure that their loved ones are protected in various situations. This proactive approach can significantly enhance the quality of life for individuals with Asperger's.

The Association for Behavior Analysis International is also instrumental in promoting evidence-based practices in the treatment of autism spectrum disorders. They emphasize the importance of applied behavior analysis (ABA) as an effective method for supporting individuals with Asperger's.

Families can explore workshops, conferences, and training sessions offered by this organization to learn more about ABA techniques and how to implement them effectively at home. This knowledge can help families implement strategies that foster positive behaviors and skills development in their loved ones.

Lastly, local and regional organizations often provide tailored support that addresses the specific needs of families in different areas. These organizations may host workshops, peer support groups, and social events that help to build a sense of community among families dealing with similar challenges.

By connecting with local groups, families can find camaraderie and support, which can be incredibly beneficial in navigating the complexities of living with and supporting a loved one with Asperger's syndrome. Engaging with professional organizations not only aids in gaining knowledge but also fosters a network of support that can make a significant difference in the lives of families.

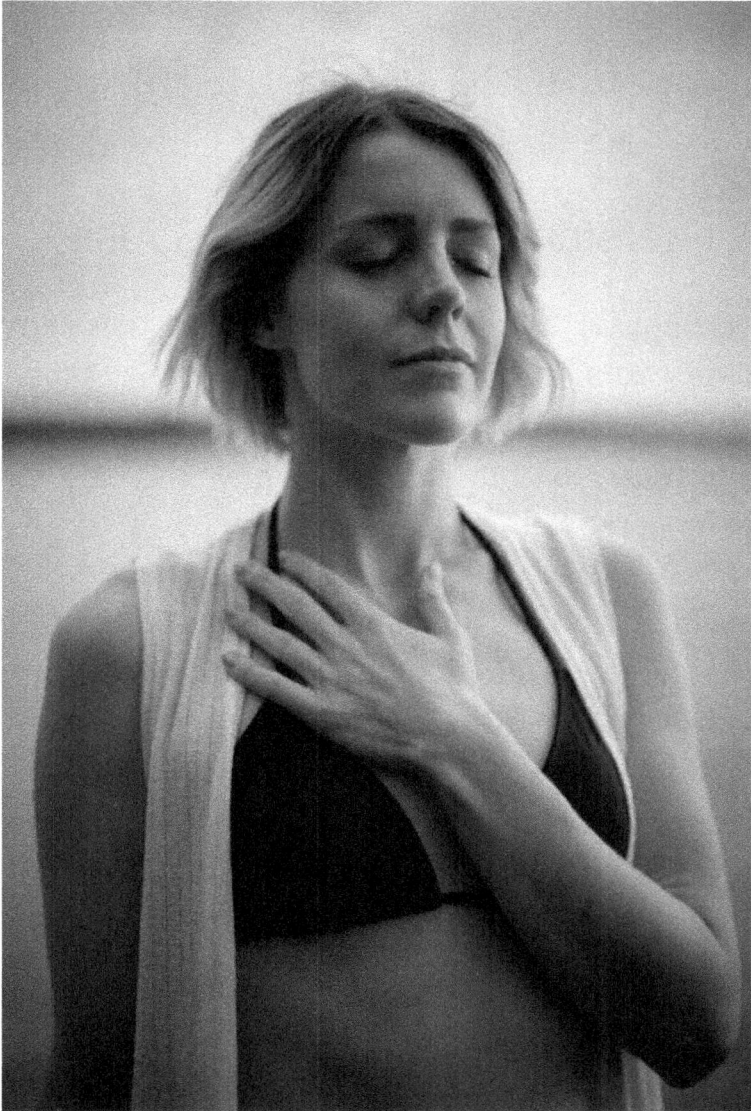

Chapter 10
Caring for Yourself

Understanding Caregiver Stress

Caregiver stress is a significant concern for families supporting loved ones with Asperger's syndrome. The unique challenges posed by this condition can lead to emotional, physical, and mental strain on caregivers.

Understanding the nature of caregiver stress is essential for developing effective coping strategies and ensuring that both the caregiver and the individual with Asperger's can thrive. Caregivers often face various pressures, including the need to advocate for their loved ones, manage daily routines, and navigate social situations that may be overwhelming for their family members.

The emotional toll of caregiving can be profound. Caregivers may experience feelings of frustration, isolation, and sadness, especially when faced with the complexities of their loved one's behavior and the societal stigma surrounding autism.

These emotions can be exacerbated by a lack of understanding from friends and family, leading caregivers to feel unsupported. It is crucial for caregivers to acknowledge their feelings and recognize that experiencing stress is a normal response to the demanding role they play.

Physical health can also be impacted by caregiver stress. Many caregivers neglect their own well-being as they prioritize the needs of their loved ones. This neglect can lead to exhaustion, sleep disturbances, and even chronic health issues over time.

Caregivers should be aware of the importance of self-care and make a conscious effort to incorporate healthy habits into their daily routines. Simple practices such as regular exercise, proper nutrition, and sufficient rest can help maintain physical health and resilience.

Mental health is another critical aspect affected by caregiver stress. Anxiety and depression are common among caregivers, particularly when they feel overwhelmed by their responsibilities. It is essential for caregivers to seek support, whether through professional counseling or support groups, where they can connect with others facing similar challenges.

Sharing experiences and coping strategies can foster a sense of community and reduce feelings of isolation, ultimately benefiting both the caregiver and the individual with Asperger's.

Recognizing and addressing caregiver stress is vital for the well-being of both parties involved. By understanding the signs of stress and taking proactive steps to manage it, caregivers can create a healthier environment for themselves and their loved ones. This includes setting realistic expectations, seeking help when needed, and allowing themselves the grace to rest and recharge. Supporting a loved one with Asperger's can be demanding, but with the right strategies in place, caregivers can sustain their energy and compassion, fostering a stronger relationship and a more positive home environment.

Self-Care Strategies

Self-care is an essential practice for family members caring for a loved one with Asperger's. It is vital to recognize that supporting someone with Asperger's can be emotionally and physically demanding. Therefore, prioritizing self-care not only benefits the caregiver but also positively impacts the relationship with the loved one.

By investing time and energy into their own well-being, caregivers can maintain their resilience and capacity to provide effective support.

One effective self-care strategy is establishing clear boundaries. Caregivers often find themselves overwhelmed by the needs of their loved ones, leading to burnout. Setting boundaries helps define the limits of what one can reasonably offer without sacrificing personal health and happiness. This can involve designated times for caregiving and personal time to recharge. Communicating these boundaries clearly and compassionately to the loved one can foster understanding and respect, ultimately contributing to a healthier dynamic.

Engaging in regular physical activity is another crucial aspect of self-care. Exercise is known to reduce stress and improve overall mental health. Caregivers should find activities that they enjoy, whether it's walking, yoga, swimming, or joining a fitness class. Incorporating physical activity into their routine can serve as a healthy outlet for stress and frustration, enhancing emotional resilience. Even short bursts of physical movement throughout the day can make a significant difference in mood and energy levels.

Mindfulness and relaxation techniques can also serve as valuable self-care strategies. Practices such as meditation, deep breathing exercises, or journaling can help caregivers process their emotions and manage anxiety. Taking a few moments each day to engage in mindfulness can create a sense of calm and clarity, enabling caregivers to approach challenges with a more balanced mindset.

Additionally, participating in support groups can provide a sense of community and shared experience, allowing caregivers to express their feelings and gain insights from others in similar situations.

Lastly, seeking professional help when needed is a crucial component of self-care. Caregivers should not hesitate to reach out to therapists or counselors who specialize in family dynamics and caregiving issues. Professional guidance can offer coping strategies and tools tailored to individual circumstances, fostering emotional health and resilience.

By prioritizing their own mental health, caregivers can create a more supportive environment for their loved ones with Asperger's, ultimately enhancing the quality of life for both parties involved.

Seeking Support for Caregivers

Caregivers of individuals with Asperger's often face unique challenges that can lead to feelings of isolation and stress. Seeking support is crucial for maintaining both the caregiver's well-being and the quality of care provided to their loved ones.

This support can take many forms, from professional resources to informal networks of friends and family. Understanding the types of support available and how to access them can greatly enhance the caregiver's experience and effectiveness.

One of the primary sources of support for caregivers is professional organizations and services. Many communities have local or national autism support organizations that provide resources, information, and networking opportunities. These organizations often host workshops, seminars, and support groups where caregivers can connect with others facing similar challenges.

Engaging with these communities can provide valuable insights and strategies, as well as emotional support. It's important for caregivers to actively seek out these resources and participate in activities that resonate with their needs.

Peer support groups can also play a significant role in alleviating the sense of loneliness that many caregivers experience. These groups offer a safe space for sharing experiences, discussing concerns, and exchanging tips on caregiving. Connecting with others who understand the unique dynamics of caring for a loved one with Asperger's can foster a sense of belonging and validation.

Many caregivers find comfort in knowing they are not alone and that their feelings are shared by others. These interactions can also lead to lasting friendships and support networks.

In addition to formal and peer support, caregivers should not underestimate the importance of seeking help from friends and family. Open communication with loved ones about the challenges faced can pave the way for practical assistance. Whether it's asking for help with daily tasks, arranging for respite care, or simply having someone to talk to, involving friends and family can lighten the emotional load.

Educating these individuals about Asperger's can also help them understand the caregiver's situation better, making it easier for them to offer meaningful support.

Finally, self-care is an essential component of seeking support. Caregivers must prioritize their own mental and physical health to effectively support their loved ones. This may involve setting aside time for personal interests, engaging in regular exercise, or seeking professional counseling.

By taking care of themselves, caregivers can maintain the energy and resilience needed to provide the best care possible. Recognizing that seeking support is not a sign of weakness but rather a proactive step towards well-being is vital for every caregiver's journey.

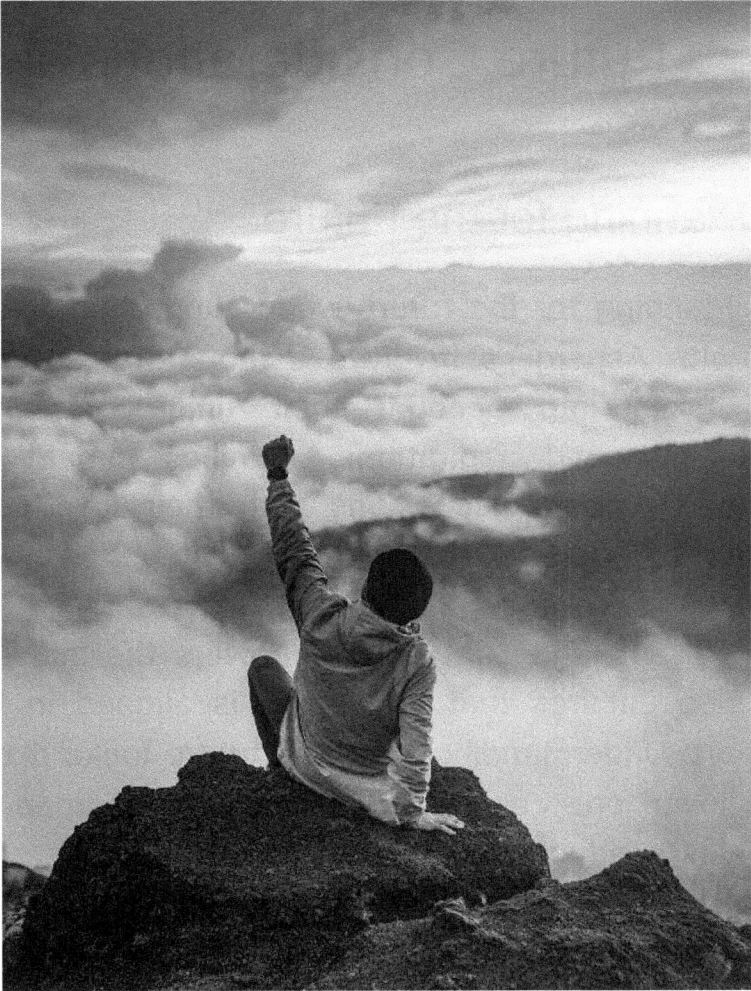

Chapter 11

Future Considerations

Planning for the Future

Planning for the future when supporting a loved one with Asperger's involves a thoughtful approach that takes into account their unique strengths, challenges, and aspirations. Families should first engage in open discussions with their loved ones about their goals and dreams.

This dialogue not only empowers the individual but also ensures that the family is aligned in their support. Understanding what the future looks like for your loved one can help you create a roadmap that includes education, employment, and social opportunities tailored to their needs.

It is crucial to consider the educational pathways available for individuals with Asperger's. Many benefit from specialized programs that focus on their learning styles and social skills development. Families should research local schools, vocational programs, and community colleges that offer supportive environments. Collaboration with educators and support staff can help in creating an Individualized Education Plan (IEP) that addresses academic and social aspects, setting the stage for future success.

Employment is another significant aspect of future planning. Identifying job opportunities that align with your loved one's interests and strengths can lead to fulfilling career paths. Families can assist by helping their loved ones explore internships or volunteer opportunities that provide real-world experience.

Networking within the community and reaching out to organizations that specialize in employment for individuals with autism can be beneficial. Encouraging your loved one to develop job skills and independence will prepare them for the workforce.

Social relationships and community involvement are vital components of a fulfilling life. Families should encourage participation in social groups, clubs, or activities that match their loved one's interests. Building social skills can take time, but with patience and encouragement, your loved one can develop meaningful connections. Planning for future social interactions not only enhances their quality of life but also provides a support network that can be invaluable in times of need.

Finally, families should consider long-term care and support strategies, especially as their loved one transitions into adulthood. Establishing legal and financial plans, including guardianship or power of attorney if needed, is essential for ensuring their well-being.

Regular family meetings to review and adjust these plans can help ensure that support remains relevant and effective. By proactively planning for the future, families can create a supportive environment that fosters independence and growth for their loved ones with Asperger's.

Long-Term Support Strategies

Long-term support strategies for individuals with Asperger's require a multifaceted approach that encompasses emotional, social, and practical considerations. Understanding the unique challenges faced by loved ones with Asperger's is essential in developing effective support systems.

Families should prioritize consistent communication to foster an environment where feelings and experiences can be shared openly. This ongoing dialogue helps to strengthen relationships and provides individuals with Asperger's the reassurance that they are understood and valued.

One crucial element of long-term support is the establishment of routines. Predictability can greatly benefit individuals with Asperger's, as it provides a sense of security and reduces anxiety. Families can collaborate to create daily and weekly schedules that outline activities, responsibilities, and downtime. Visual aids, such as charts or calendars, can assist in making these routines clear and accessible.

Flexibility within these routines is also important, allowing for adjustments based on the individual's needs and preferences while maintaining a sense of order.

Encouraging social skills development is another vital strategy. Individuals with Asperger's may struggle with social interactions, making it essential for families to provide opportunities for socialization in low-pressure environments.

Engaging in group activities, clubs, or classes tailored to their interests can help build confidence and improve social skills. Role-playing different social scenarios at home can also be beneficial, allowing loved ones to practice and refine their interactions in a safe space.

Emotional support plays a significant role in the long-term well-being of individuals with Asperger's. Families should strive to create a nurturing atmosphere where emotions can be expressed without fear of judgment. This involves recognizing and validating feelings, even when they may not fully align with societal norms.

Encouraging the use of coping strategies, such as mindfulness or journaling, can help individuals manage their emotions more effectively. Additionally, seeking professional support from therapists or counselors who specialize in Asperger's can provide further guidance and resources.

Finally, staying informed about Asperger's and related resources is essential for families supporting a loved one. Continuous education about the condition can empower families to better understand the challenges and strengths associated with Asperger's.

Attending workshops, reading literature, and connecting with other families facing similar experiences can provide valuable insights and strategies. By remaining engaged and informed, families can adapt their support strategies as their loved one grows and changes, ensuring a lasting and positive impact on their quality of life.

Celebrating Progress and Achievements

Celebrating progress and achievements is a vital aspect of supporting a loved one with Asperger's. Recognizing milestones, no matter how small, can foster a sense of accomplishment and motivation for both the individual and their support network. It is essential to create an environment where successes are acknowledged, as this reinforces positive behavior and encourages the pursuit of further goals.

Whether it is mastering a new skill, overcoming a challenge, or simply completing daily tasks, celebrating these moments can significantly enhance the individual's self-esteem and sense of belonging.

One effective way to celebrate achievements is through personalized recognition. This could involve creating a visual chart to track progress in specific areas, such as social skills or academic performance. Each time a milestone is reached, a mark or sticker can be added, which visually represents the journey taken.

This not only provides a tangible reminder of progress but also allows the individual to see their efforts culminate in visible results.

Additionally, discussing these achievements during family gatherings or special occasions can help reinforce their importance and encourage a supportive dialogue around growth and development.

Another method to celebrate progress is by incorporating rewards that align with the interests of the individual. For instance, if your loved one enjoys a particular hobby or activity, consider rewarding their achievements with something related to that interest. This could be a new book, a ticket to a special event, or even a day out doing something they love.

Tailoring rewards to their preferences ensures that the celebration feels meaningful and personal. It also helps to establish a positive association with effort and accomplishment, making the individual more likely to strive for future successes.

Moreover, it is crucial to involve your loved one in the celebration process. Encourage them to reflect on their achievements and express how they feel about them. This can be done through discussions or creative outlets, such as journaling or art.

By allowing them to articulate their feelings about their progress, you not only validate their experiences but also empower them to take ownership of their achievements. This practice can help develop self-awareness and encourage a proactive approach to future challenges.

Finally, celebrating progress should not be limited to significant milestones. It is important to recognize day-to-day achievements, such as completing a challenging task or effectively communicating a need. These celebrations can be as simple as verbal praise or small gestures of encouragement. Consistently acknowledging these moments cultivates a positive atmosphere where your loved one feels valued and supported.

By making celebration a regular practice, you contribute to a nurturing environment that promotes continued growth and resilience.

Author Notes & Acknowledgments

First and foremost, I would like to express my deepest gratitude to the people who inspired and supported me throughout the journey of writing this book. This project would not have been possible without their unwavering belief in me and their invaluable contributions.

To my wife, thank you for your constant encouragement and understanding. Your love and support have been my anchor during the challenging times of researching and writing this book. Your belief in my ability to make a difference in people's lives has been my driving force.

I would also like to disclose that this book contains some renewed artificial intelligence-generated content. I really appreciate very recent technological innovation by outstanding scientists and of course our reader's understanding.

Lastly, I want to express my deepest gratitude to the readers of this book. I sincerely hope the strategies and methods outlined within these pages will provide you with the knowledge and tools needed to truly make your life much better. Your commitment to seeking any good solutions and willingness to explore multiple methods is commendable.

Author Bio

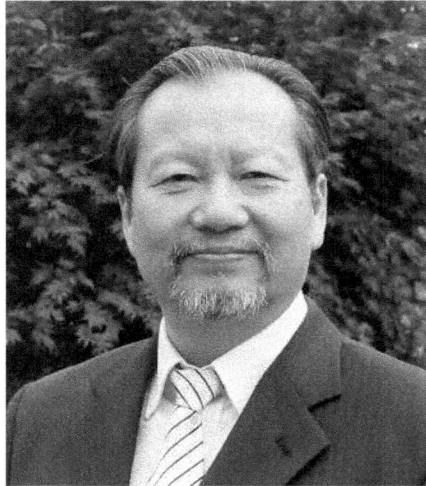

Johnson Wu earned his MD in 1982. With over 40 years of clinical experience, he has worked in hospitals in Zhejiang and Shanghai, China, as well as the Royal Marsden Hospital (part of Imperial College) in London, UK. Upon the recommendation of Sir Aaron Klug, the president of The Royal Society and a Nobel Prize winner in Chemistry, Dr. Wu was honorably awarded a British Royal Society Fellowship. He has published over 100 medical books in many countries and currently practices medicine in Canada.

www.ingramcontent.com/pod-product-compliance
Lightning Source LLC
Chambersburg PA
CBHW060240030426

42335CB00014B/1555